Date: _____ Patient Name: _____

APPOINTMENT: _____

Patient Details:

_____

_____

_____

```
||| ||| || ||| ||| |||
G000066192
```

Patient Histry:

_____

_____

_____

| SYMPTOMS | MEDICATION | CONCERNS |
|---|---|---|
|  |  |  |

My Thoughts and notes

_____

_____

_____

Future Check Up's

_____

_____

IMPORTANT

_____

_____

Date:_____ Patient Name: _____

APPOINTMENT: _____

## Patient Details:
_____
_____
_____
_____

## Patient Histry:
_____
_____
_____
_____

| SYMPTOMS | MEDICATION | CONCERNS |
|---|---|---|
|  |  |  |

### My Thoughts and notes

Future Check Up's

_____
_____
_____

### IMPORTANT
_____
_____
_____

Date: _____ Patient Name: _____

APPOINTMENT: _____

## Patient Details:
_____
_____
_____
_____

## Patient Histry:
_____
_____
_____
_____

| SYMPTOMS | MEDICATION | CONCERNS |
|---|---|---|
| | | |

### My Thoughts and notes

### Future Check Up's
_____
_____
_____

_____
_____
_____

### IMPORTANT
_____
_____
_____

Date: _____ Patient Name: _____

APPOINTMENT: _____

## Patient Details:
_____
_____
_____
_____

## Patient Histry:
_____
_____
_____
_____

| SYMPTOMS | MEDICATION | CONCERNS |
|---|---|---|
| | | |

### My Thoughts and notes

Future Check Up's

_____
_____
_____

IMPORTANT

_____
_____
_____

Date:_____ Patient Name:_____

APPOINTMENT: _____

## Patient Details:

_____
_____
_____
_____

## Patient Histry:

_____
_____
_____
_____

| SYMPTOMS | MEDICATION | CONCERNS |
|---|---|---|
|  |  |  |

### My Thoughts and notes

_____
_____
_____
_____

### Future Check Up's

_____
_____

**IMPORTANT**

_____
_____
_____

Date: ~~THERSDAY~~ Patient Name: LUNA

APPOINTMENT: 

## Patient Details:
~~BROCEN PAW AND~~
~~BROWKEN EAR~~

## Patient Histry:
~~Broke paw by dog fight~~
~~broke ear by dog fight~~

| SYMPTOMS | MEDICATION | CONCERNS |
|----------|------------|----------|
|          |            |          |

My Thoughts and notes

Future Check Up's

IMPORTANT

Date: **thursday 7 7**   Patient Name: **leo**

APPOINTMENT: _____

## Patient Details:
tail Brocken
_____
_____

## Patient Histry:
he Brocke in ruff and tample
time at puppy class

| SYMPTOMS | MEDICATION | CONCERNS |
|---|---|---|
|  |  |  |

My Thoughts and notes

Future Check Up's

IMPORTANT

Date:_____ Patient Name: _____

APPOINTMENT: _____

## Patient Details:

_____
_____
_____
_____

## Patient Histry:

_____
_____
_____
_____
_____

| SYMPTOMS | MEDICATION | CONCERNS |
|---|---|---|
|  |  |  |

### My Thoughts and notes

### Future Check Up's

_____
_____
_____
_____

_____

IMPORTANT

_____
_____

Date:_____ Patient Name:_____

APPOINTMENT: _____

Patient Details:
_____
_____
_____

Patient Histry:
_____
_____
_____
_____

| SYMPTOMS | MEDICATION | CONCERNS |
|---|---|---|
|  |  |  |

My Thoughts and notes

Future Check Up's
_____
_____
_____

_____
_____
_____

IMPORTANT
_____
_____

Date:_____ Patient Name:_____

APPOINTMENT: _____

Patient Details:
_____
_____
_____
_____

Patient Histry:
_____
_____
_____
_____

| SYMPTOMS | MEDICATION | CONCERNS |
|----------|------------|----------|
|          |            |          |

My Thoughts and notes

Future Check Up's

IMPORTANT

Date:_____ Patient Name:_____

APPOINTMENT: _____

## Patient Details:
_____
_____
_____
_____

## Patient Histry:
_____
_____
_____
_____
_____

| SYMPTOMS | MEDICATION | CONCERNS |
|---|---|---|

*My Thoughts and notes*

*Future Check Up's*

_____ _____
_____ _____
_____
_____
_____

IMPORTANT

_____
_____

Date:_____ Patient Name:_____

APPOINTMENT: _____

# Patient Details:

_____
_____
_____
_____

# Patient Histry:

_____
_____
_____
_____
_____

| SYMPTOMS | MEDICATION | CONCERNS |
|----------|------------|----------|
|          |            |          |

## My Thoughts and notes

Future Check Up's

_____
_____
_____
_____

### IMPORTANT

_____
_____
_____

Date:_____ Patient Name:_____

APPOINTMENT: _____

## Patient Details:

_____
_____
_____
_____

## Patient Histry:

_____
_____
_____
_____
_____

| SYMPTOMS | MEDICATION | CONCERNS |
|----------|------------|----------|
|          |            |          |

My Thoughts and notes          Future Check Up's

_____          _____
_____
_____          _____
_____

IMPORTANT

_____
_____
_____

Date:_____ Patient Name:_____

APPOINTMENT: _____

## Patient Details:
_____
_____
_____
_____

## Patient Histry:
_____
_____
_____
_____

| SYMPTOMS | MEDICATION | CONCERNS |
|---|---|---|
|  |  |  |

### My Thoughts and notes
_____
_____
_____
_____

### Future Check Up's
_____
_____
_____

IMPORTANT
_____
_____
_____

Date:_____ Patient Name:_____

APPOINTMENT: _____

## Patient Details:
_____
_____
_____
_____

## Patient Histry:
_____
_____
_____
_____

| SYMPTOMS | MEDICATION | CONCERNS |
|---|---|---|
|  |  |  |

### My Thoughts and notes
_____

### Future Check Up's
_____
_____

### IMPORTANT
_____

Date:_____ Patient Name:_____

APPOINTMENT: _____

## Patient Details:

_____
_____
_____
_____

## Patient Histry:

_____
_____
_____
_____
_____

| SYMPTOMS | MEDICATION | CONCERNS |
|----------|------------|----------|
|          |            |          |

### My Thoughts and notes

Future Check Up's

_____
_____          _____
_____          _____
_____

### IMPORTANT

_____
_____
_____

Date: _____ Patient Name: _____

APPOINTMENT: _____

## Patient Details:
_____
_____
_____
_____

## Patient Histry:
_____
_____
_____
_____

| SYMPTOMS | MEDICATION | CONCERNS |
|---|---|---|
| | | |

*My Thoughts and notes*

*Future Check Up's*

_____
_____
_____

**IMPORTANT**

_____
_____
_____

Date: _____ Patient Name: _____

APPOINTMENT: _____

## Patient Details:

_____
_____
_____

## Patient Histry:

_____
_____
_____
_____

| SYMPTOMS | MEDICATION | CONCERNS |
|---|---|---|
|  |  |  |

My Thoughts and notes

Future Check Up's

_____
_____
_____

IMPORTANT

Date:_____ Patient Name:_____

APPOINTMENT: _____

## Patient Details:

_____
_____
_____
_____

## Patient Histry:

_____
_____
_____
_____

| SYMPTOMS | MEDICATION | CONCERNS |
|---|---|---|
|  |  |  |

## My Thoughts and notes

Future Check Up's

_____
_____
_____

IMPORTANT

_____
_____

Date:_____ Patient Name:_____

APPOINTMENT: _____

## Patient Details:
_____
_____
_____
_____

## Patient Histry:
_____
_____
_____
_____
_____

| SYMPTOMS | MEDICATION | CONCERNS |
|---|---|---|
|  |  |  |

### My Thoughts and notes

Future Check Up's

_____
_____
_____
_____

### IMPORTANT
_____
_____
_____

Date:_____ Patient Name:_____

APPOINTMENT: _____

## Patient Details:
_____
_____
_____
_____

## Patient Histry:
_____
_____
_____
_____

| SYMPTOMS | MEDICATION | CONCERNS |
|---|---|---|
| | | |

My Thoughts and notes

Future Check Up's

_____    _____
_____
_____    _____

IMPORTANT
_____
_____
_____

Date:_____ Patient Name:_____

APPOINTMENT: _____

## Patient Details:
_____
_____
_____
_____

## Patient Histry:
_____
_____
_____
_____
_____

| SYMPTOMS | MEDICATION | CONCERNS |
|---|---|---|
|  |  |  |

### My Thoughts and notes
_____
_____
_____

### Future Check Up's
_____
_____
_____

### IMPORTANT
_____
_____
_____

Date:_____ Patient Name:_____

APPOINTMENT: _____

## Patient Details:
_____
_____
_____
_____

## Patient Histry:
_____
_____
_____
_____

| SYMPTOMS | MEDICATION | CONCERNS |
|---|---|---|
|  |  |  |

My Thoughts and notes

Future Check Up's

_____
_____
_____

IMPORTANT

_____
_____
_____

Date:_____ Patient Name:_____

APPOINTMENT: _____

## Patient Details:
_____
_____
_____

## Patient Histry:
_____
_____
_____
_____

| SYMPTOMS | MEDICATION | CONCERNS |
|----------|------------|----------|
|          |            |          |

### My Thoughts and notes

Future Check Up's

_____

IMPORTANT

Date:_____ Patient Name:_____

APPOINTMENT: _____

## Patient Details:
_____
_____
_____
_____

## Patient Histry:
_____
_____
_____
_____

| SYMPTOMS | MEDICATION | CONCERNS |
|---|---|---|
|  |  |  |

My Thoughts and notes

Future Check Up's

_____
_____
_____

IMPORTANT

_____
_____
_____

Date:_____ Patient Name:_____

APPOINTMENT: _____

## Patient Details:
_____
_____
_____
_____

## Patient Histry:
_____
_____
_____
_____

| SYMPTOMS | MEDICATION | CONCERNS |
|---|---|---|
|  |  |  |

My Thoughts and notes

Future Check Up's

_____
_____
_____

IMPORTANT
_____
_____
_____

Date:_____ Patient Name:_____

APPOINTMENT: _____

## Patient Details:
_____
_____
_____
_____

## Patient Histry:
_____
_____
_____
_____
_____

| SYMPTOMS | MEDICATION | CONCERNS |
|----------|------------|----------|
|          |            |          |

### My Thoughts and notes
_____
_____
_____

Future Check Up's
_____
_____

IMPORTANT
_____
_____
_____

Date:_____ Patient Name: _____

APPOINTMENT: _____

## Patient Details:
_____
_____
_____
_____

## Patient Histry:
_____
_____
_____
_____
_____

| SYMPTOMS | MEDICATION | CONCERNS |
|----------|------------|----------|
|          |            |          |

### My Thoughts and notes

Future Check Up's

_____
_____

#### IMPORTANT

BIRTHDAY WEEK

**Date:** TUESDAY  **Patient Name:** ROSE MORLEY

APPOINTMENT: QWARTER TO 4

## Patient Details:
GOT CORONER VIRES

## Patient Histry:
APSOLOLY FEELFINE MIGHT HAVE GOT
IT FROMBUS OR SOPHIA

| SYMPTOMS | MEDICATION | CONCERNS |
|---|---|---|
| EYES STING | NO MEDSON YET | I FEEL SICK EVERY NOW AND THEN |

## My Thoughts and notes

## Future Check Up's

## IMPORTANT

# Date: _____ Patient Name: _____

APPOINTMENT: _____

## Patient Details:

_____
_____
_____
_____

## Patient Histry:

_____
_____
_____
_____

| SYMPTOMS | MEDICATION | CONCERNS |
|----------|------------|----------|
|          |            |          |

## My Thoughts and notes

### Future Check Up's

_____
_____
_____

### IMPORTANT

_____

Date:_____ Patient Name:_____

APPOINTMENT: _____

## Patient Details:
_____
_____
_____
_____

## Patient Histry:
_____
_____
_____
_____

| SYMPTOMS | MEDICATION | CONCERNS |
|----------|------------|----------|
|          |            |          |

### My Thoughts and notes
_____
_____
_____

### Future Check Up's
_____
_____

### IMPORTANT
_____
_____
_____

Date:_____ Patient Name:_____

APPOINTMENT: _____

## Patient Details:

_____
_____
_____
_____

## Patient Histry:

_____
_____
_____
_____

| SYMPTOMS | MEDICATION | CONCERNS |
|---|---|---|
|  |  |  |

My Thoughts and notes        Future Check Up's

_____          _____
_____          _____
_____          _____
_____

IMPORTANT

_____
_____
_____

Date:_____ Patient Name:_____

APPOINTMENT: _____

## Patient Details:

_____
_____
_____
_____

## Patient Histry:

_____
_____
_____
_____

| SYMPTOMS | MEDICATION | CONCERNS |
|----------|------------|----------|
|          |            |          |

My Thoughts and notes

Future Check Up's

_____    _____
_____    _____
_____

IMPORTANT

_____
_____
_____

Date:_____ Patient Name: _____

APPOINTMENT: _____

## Patient Details:

_____
_____
_____
_____

## Patient Histry:

_____
_____
_____
_____

| SYMPTOMS | MEDICATION | CONCERNS |
|----------|------------|----------|
|          |            |          |

My Thoughts and notes                    Future Check Up's

_____          _____
_____          _____
_____          _____

IMPORTANT

_____
_____
_____

Date:_____ Patient Name:_____

APPOINTMENT: _____

Patient Details:
_____
_____
_____
_____

Patient Histry:
_____
_____
_____
_____

| SYMPTOMS | MEDICATION | CONCERNS |
|---|---|---|

My Thoughts and notes
_____
_____
_____

Future Check Up's
_____
_____

IMPORTANT
_____
_____

Date:_____ Patient Name:_____

APPOINTMENT: _____

## Patient Details:
_____
_____
_____
_____

## Patient Histry:
_____
_____
_____
_____
_____

| SYMPTOMS | MEDICATION | CONCERNS |
|---|---|---|
| | | |

### My Thoughts and notes
_____
_____
_____
_____

#### Future Check Up's
_____
_____

### IMPORTANT
_____
_____
_____

Date: _____ Patient Name: _____

APPOINTMENT: _____

## Patient Details:
_____
_____
_____
_____

## Patient Histry:
_____
_____
_____
_____
_____

| SYMPTOMS | MEDICATION | CONCERNS |
|---|---|---|
|  |  |  |

### My Thoughts and notes
_____
_____
_____

### Future Check Up's
_____
_____

IMPORTANT
_____
_____

Date: _____ Patient Name: _____

APPOINTMENT: _____

## Patient Details:

_____
_____
_____

## Patient Histry:

_____
_____
_____
_____

| SYMPTOMS | MEDICATION | CONCERNS |
|----------|------------|----------|
|          |            |          |

### My Thoughts and notes

_____
_____
_____

### Future Check Up's

_____
_____

### IMPORTANT

_____
_____
_____

**Date:** _____ **Patient Name:** _____

APPOINTMENT: _____

## Patient Details:

_____
_____
_____
_____

## Patient Histry:

_____
_____
_____
_____
_____

| SYMPTOMS | MEDICATION | CONCERNS |
|----------|------------|----------|
|          |            |          |

### My Thoughts and notes

_____
_____
_____

### Future Check Up's

.......................
.......................

### IMPORTANT

_____
_____
_____

Date:_____ Patient Name:_____

APPOINTMENT: _____

Patient Details:
_____
_____
_____
_____

Patient Histry:
_____
_____
_____
_____
_____

| SYMPTOMS | MEDICATION | CONCERNS |
|---|---|---|
|  |  |  |

My Thoughts and notes

Future Check Up's

IMPORTANT

Date: _____ Patient Name: _____

APPOINTMENT: _____

## Patient Details:

_____
_____
_____
_____

## Patient Histry:

_____
_____
_____
_____
_____

| SYMPTOMS | MEDICATION | CONCERNS |
|---|---|---|
| | | |

### My Thoughts and notes

_____

Future Check Up's

_____

### IMPORTANT

_____

Date:_____ Patient Name:_____

APPOINTMENT: _____

## Patient Details:

_____
_____
_____

## Patient Histry:

_____
_____
_____
_____

| SYMPTOMS | MEDICATION | CONCERNS |
|----------|------------|----------|
|          |            |          |

### My Thoughts and notes

_____
_____
_____
_____

### IMPORTANT

_____
_____
_____

### Future Check Up's

_____
_____
_____

Date:_____ Patient Name:_____

APPOINTMENT: _____

## Patient Details:

_____
_____
_____
_____

## Patient Histry:

_____
_____
_____
_____

| SYMPTOMS | MEDICATION | CONCERNS |
|---|---|---|
|  |  |  |

My Thoughts and notes

Future Check Up's

_____          _____
_____          _____
_____          _____

IMPORTANT

_____
_____
_____

# Date: _____ Patient Name: _____

APPOINTMENT: _____

## Patient Details:
_____
_____
_____

## Patient Histry:
_____
_____
_____

| SYMPTOMS | MEDICATION | CONCERNS |
|----------|------------|----------|
|          |            |          |

### My Thoughts and notes

_____
_____
_____

### Future Check Up's
_____
_____
_____

### IMPORTANT
_____
_____

Date:_____ Patient Name:_____

APPOINTMENT: _____

## Patient Details:
_____
_____
_____
_____

## Patient Histry:
_____
_____
_____
_____

| SYMPTOMS | MEDICATION | CONCERNS |
|---|---|---|
|  |  |  |

### My Thoughts and notes
_____
_____
_____
_____

### Future Check Up's
_____
_____

### IMPORTANT
_____
_____
_____

Date:_____ Patient Name:_____

APPOINTMENT: _____

## Patient Details:
_____
_____
_____
_____

## Patient Histry:
_____
_____
_____
_____

| SYMPTOMS | MEDICATION | CONCERNS |
|----------|------------|----------|
|          |            |          |

### My Thoughts and notes

_____
_____
_____

### IMPORTANT

_____
_____
_____

### Future Check Up's
_____
_____
_____

Date:_____ Patient Name:_____

APPOINTMENT: _____

## Patient Details:
_____
_____
_____

## Patient Histry:
_____
_____
_____

| SYMPTOMS | MEDICATION | CONCERNS |
|---|---|---|
| | | |

### My Thoughts and notes
_____
_____

**Future Check Up's**
_____
_____

### IMPORTANT
_____
_____

Date:_____ Patient Name:_____

APPOINTMENT: _____

## Patient Details:
_____
_____
_____
_____

## Patient Histry:
_____
_____
_____
_____
_____

| SYMPTOMS | MEDICATION | CONCERNS |
|---|---|---|
|  |  |  |

My Thoughts and notes

Future Check Up's

_____
_____
_____
_____

IMPORTANT

_____
_____

Date:_____ Patient Name:_____

APPOINTMENT: _____

## Patient Details:

_____
_____
_____
_____

## Patient Histry:

_____
_____
_____
_____

| SYMPTOMS | MEDICATION | CONCERNS |
|----------|------------|----------|
|          |            |          |

### My Thoughts and notes

_____

### Future Check Up's

_____

### IMPORTANT

_____

Date:_____ Patient Name:_____

APPOINTMENT: _____

## Patient Details:

_____
_____
_____
_____

## Patient Histry:

_____
_____
_____
_____

| SYMPTOMS | MEDICATION | CONCERNS |
|----------|------------|----------|
|          |            |          |

### My Thoughts and notes

Future Check Up's

_____       _____
_____       _____
_____       _____
_____

### IMPORTANT

_____
_____
_____

Date:_____ Patient Name:_____

APPOINTMENT: _____

## Patient Details:
_____
_____
_____
_____

## Patient Histry:
_____
_____
_____
_____

| SYMPTOMS | MEDICATION | CONCERNS |
|----------|------------|----------|
|          |            |          |

My Thoughts and notes

Future Check Up's

_____
_____
_____

IMPORTANT
_____
_____
_____

Date:_____ Patient Name:_____

APPOINTMENT: _____

## Patient Details:

_____
_____
_____
_____

## Patient Histry:

_____
_____
_____
_____

| SYMPTOMS | MEDICATION | CONCERNS |
|---|---|---|
| | | |

### My Thoughts and notes

_____
_____
_____

### Future Check Up's

_____
_____
_____

IMPORTANT

_____
_____
_____

Date:_____ Patient Name: _____

APPOINTMENT: _____

# Patient Details:

_____
_____
_____
_____

# Patient Histry:

_____
_____
_____
_____

| SYMPTOMS | MEDICATION | CONCERNS |
|---|---|---|
| | | |

## My Thoughts and notes

_____

_____

_____

### IMPORTANT

_____

_____

## Future Check Up's

_____

_____

Date:_____ Patient Name:_____

APPOINTMENT: _____

## Patient Details:
_____
_____
_____

## Patient Histry:
_____
_____
_____
_____

| SYMPTOMS | MEDICATION | CONCERNS |
|----------|------------|----------|
|          |            |          |

My Thoughts and notes          Future Check Up's
_____    _____
_____    _____
_____    _____

IMPORTANT
_____
_____
_____

Date:_____ Patient Name:_____

APPOINTMENT: _____

## Patient Details:
_____
_____
_____
_____

## Patient Histry:
_____
_____
_____
_____

| SYMPTOMS | MEDICATION | CONCERNS |
|---|---|---|
|  |  |  |

### My Thoughts and notes

### Future Check Up's

_____
_____
_____
_____

### IMPORTANT
_____
_____
_____

Date:_____ Patient Name: _____

APPOINTMENT: _____

## Patient Details:

_____
_____
_____
_____

## Patient Histry:

_____
_____
_____
_____
_____
_____

| SYMPTOMS | MEDICATION | CONCERNS |
|----------|------------|----------|
|          |            |          |

My Thoughts and notes

Future Check Up's

IMPORTANT

# Date:_____ Patient Name:_____

APPOINTMENT: _____

## Patient Details:
_____
_____
_____
_____

## Patient Histry:
_____
_____
_____
_____
_____

| SYMPTOMS | MEDICATION | CONCERNS |
|----------|------------|----------|
|          |            |          |

## My Thoughts and notes

Future Check Up's

_____
_____
_____
_____

### IMPORTANT
_____
_____

Date: _____ Patient Name: _____

APPOINTMENT: _____

Patient Details:
_____
_____
_____
_____

Patient Histry:
_____
_____
_____
_____

| SYMPTOMS | MEDICATION | CONCERNS |
|---|---|---|

My Thoughts and notes

Future Check Up's

_____
_____
_____

IMPORTANT
_____
_____
_____

Date:_____ Patient Name:_____

APPOINTMENT: _____

## Patient Details:
_____
_____
_____
_____

## Patient Histry:
_____
_____
_____
_____
_____

| SYMPTOMS | MEDICATION | CONCERNS |
|---|---|---|
| | | |

## My Thoughts and notes

Future Check Up's

_____
_____
_____
_____

### IMPORTANT

_____
_____
_____

Date: _____ Patient Name: _____

APPOINTMENT: _____

## Patient Details:
_____
_____
_____
_____

## Patient Histry:
_____
_____
_____
_____
_____

| SYMPTOMS | MEDICATION | CONCERNS |
|----------|------------|----------|
|          |            |          |

### My Thoughts and notes

Future Check Up's

_____
_____
_____

#### IMPORTANT

_____
_____
_____

Date:_____ Patient Name:_____

APPOINTMENT: _____

## Patient Details:

_____
_____
_____
_____

## Patient Histry:

_____
_____
_____
_____
_____

| SYMPTOMS | MEDICATION | CONCERNS |
|---|---|---|
|  |  |  |

### My Thoughts and notes

_____

### Future Check Up's

_____

#### IMPORTANT

Date:_____ Patient Name:_____

APPOINTMENT: _____

## Patient Details:

_____
_____
_____

## Patient Histry:

_____
_____
_____
_____

| SYMPTOMS | MEDICATION | CONCERNS |
|---|---|---|
|  |  |  |

### My Thoughts and notes

_____
_____
_____

### Future Check Up's

_____

### IMPORTANT

_____
_____
_____

Date:_____ Patient Name: _____

APPOINTMENT: _____

## Patient Details:

_____
_____
_____
_____

## Patient Histry:

_____
_____
_____
_____

| SYMPTOMS | MEDICATION | CONCERNS |
|----------|------------|----------|
|          |            |          |

### My Thoughts and notes

_____
_____
_____

### Future Check Up's

_____
_____

**IMPORTANT**

_____
_____
_____

Date:_____ Patient Name: _____

APPOINTMENT: _____

## Patient Details:

_____
_____
_____

## Patient Histry:

_____
_____
_____

| SYMPTOMS | MEDICATION | CONCERNS |
|----------|------------|----------|
|          |            |          |

My Thoughts and notes

Future Check Up's

_____
_____
_____

IMPORTANT

_____
_____

Date:_____ Patient Name:_____

APPOINTMENT: _____

## Patient Details:
_____
_____
_____

## Patient Histry:
_____
_____
_____
_____

| SYMPTOMS | MEDICATION | CONCERNS |
|----------|------------|----------|
|          |            |          |

### My Thoughts and notes

_____
_____
_____

### IMPORTANT

_____
_____

### Future Check Up's
_____
_____
_____

Date:_____ Patient Name:_____

APPOINTMENT: _____

Patient Details:
_____
_____
_____
_____

Patient Histry:
_____
_____
_____
_____
_____

| SYMPTOMS | MEDICATION | CONCERNS |
|----------|------------|----------|
|          |            |          |

My Thoughts and notes

Future Check Up's

_____
_____
_____
_____

IMPORTANT

_____
_____
_____

Date:_____ Patient Name:_____

APPOINTMENT: _____

## Patient Details:
_____
_____
_____
_____

## Patient Histry:
_____
_____
_____
_____
_____

| SYMPTOMS | MEDICATION | CONCERNS |
|---|---|---|
|  |  |  |

### My Thoughts and notes
_____
_____
_____

### Future Check Up's
_____
_____

### IMPORTANT
_____
_____
_____

Date: _____ Patient Name: _____

APPOINTMENT: _____

## Patient Details:
_____
_____
_____

## Patient Histry:
_____
_____
_____
_____

| SYMPTOMS | MEDICATION | CONCERNS |
|---|---|---|
|  |  |  |

### My Thoughts and notes

Future Check Up's

_____
_____
_____
_____

### IMPORTANT

_____
_____
_____

Date:_____ Patient Name:_____

APPOINTMENT: _____

## Patient Details:

_____
_____
_____
_____

## Patient Histry:

_____
_____
_____
_____

| SYMPTOMS | MEDICATION | CONCERNS |
|---|---|---|
|  |  |  |

### My Thoughts and notes

Future Check Up's

_____
_____
_____
_____

### IMPORTANT

_____
_____
_____
_____

Date:_____ Patient Name:_____

APPOINTMENT: _____

## Patient Details:
_____
_____
_____
_____

## Patient Histry:
_____
_____
_____
_____
_____

| SYMPTOMS | MEDICATION | CONCERNS |
|----------|------------|----------|
|          |            |          |

### My Thoughts and notes

### Future Check Up's

IMPORTANT

Date:_____ Patient Name:_____

APPOINTMENT: _____

## Patient Details:

_____
_____
_____
_____

## Patient Histry:

_____
_____
_____
_____

| SYMPTOMS | MEDICATION | CONCERNS |
|----------|------------|----------|
|          |            |          |

### My Thoughts and notes

_____

### Future Check Up's

_____
_____

### IMPORTANT

_____
_____

Date:_____ Patient Name:_____

APPOINTMENT: _____

## Patient Details:

_____
_____
_____

## Patient Histry:

_____
_____
_____
_____

| SYMPTOMS | MEDICATION | CONCERNS |
|----------|------------|----------|
|          |            |          |

### My Thoughts and notes

Future Check Up's

_____  ...............
_____  ...............
_____
_____

### IMPORTANT

_____
_____
_____

Date:_____ Patient Name:_____

APPOINTMENT: _____

## Patient Details:
_____
_____
_____

## Patient Histry:
_____
_____
_____

| SYMPTOMS | MEDICATION | CONCERNS |
|---|---|---|
| | | |

### My Thoughts and notes
_____
_____
_____

### Future Check Up's
_____

IMPORTANT
_____
_____

Date: _____ Patient Name: _____

APPOINTMENT: _____

# Patient Details:

_____
_____
_____
_____

# Patient Histry:

_____
_____
_____
_____

| SYMPTOMS | MEDICATION | CONCERNS |
|----------|------------|----------|
|          |            |          |

## My Thoughts and notes

Future Check Up's

_____
_____
_____

### IMPORTANT

_____
_____
_____

Date: _____ Patient Name: _____

APPOINTMENT: _____

## Patient Details:

_____
_____
_____
_____

## Patient Histry:

_____
_____
_____
_____

| SYMPTOMS | MEDICATION | CONCERNS |
|----------|-----------|----------|
|          |           |          |

## My Thoughts and notes

Future Check Up's

_____
_____
_____
_____

IMPORTANT

_____
_____

Date:_____ Patient Name:_____

APPOINTMENT: _____

Patient Details:
_____
_____
_____
_____

Patient Histry:
_____
_____
_____
_____

| SYMPTOMS | MEDICATION | CONCERNS |
|----------|------------|----------|
|          |            |          |

My Thoughts and notes

Future Check Up's

_____
_____
_____
_____

IMPORTANT

_____
_____
_____

Date:_____ Patient Name:_____

APPOINTMENT: _____

## Patient Details:

_____
_____
_____
_____

## Patient Histry:

_____
_____
_____
_____

| SYMPTOMS | MEDICATION | CONCERNS |
|---|---|---|
|  |  |  |

### My Thoughts and notes

Future Check Up's

_____  ......................
_____  ......................
_____
_____

IMPORTANT

_____
_____
_____
_____

Date:_____ Patient Name: _____

APPOINTMENT: _____

## Patient Details:

_____
_____
_____
_____

## Patient Histry:

_____
_____
_____
_____
_____

| SYMPTOMS | MEDICATION | CONCERNS |
|---|---|---|

*My Thoughts and notes*                    *Future Check Up's*

_____        ─ ─ ─ ─ ─ ─ ─
_____        ─ ─ ─ ─ ─ ─ ─
_____

**IMPORTANT**

_____
_____
_____

Date: _____ Patient Name: _____

APPOINTMENT: _____

# Patient Details:

_____
_____
_____
_____

# Patient Histry:

_____
_____
_____
_____

| SYMPTOMS | MEDICATION | CONCERNS |
|----------|------------|----------|
|          |            |          |

## My Thoughts and notes

Future Check Up's

_____
_____
_____
_____

## IMPORTANT

_____
_____
_____

Date:_____ Patient Name: _____

APPOINTMENT: _____

## Patient Details:
_____
_____
_____
_____

## Patient Histry:
_____
_____
_____
_____

| SYMPTOMS | MEDICATION | CONCERNS |
|----------|------------|----------|
|          |            |          |

### My Thoughts and notes

Future Check Up's

_____
_____
_____
_____

### IMPORTANT
_____
_____
_____

Date:_____ Patient Name:_____

APPOINTMENT: _____

## Patient Details:

_____
_____
_____
_____

## Patient Histry:

_____
_____
_____
_____

| SYMPTOMS | MEDICATION | CONCERNS |
|----------|------------|----------|
|          |            |          |

### My Thoughts and notes

Future Check Up's

_____
_____
_____
_____

**IMPORTANT**

_____
_____
_____

Date:_____ Patient Name:_____

APPOINTMENT: _____

## Patient Details:

_____
_____
_____
_____

## Patient Histry:

_____
_____
_____
_____

| SYMPTOMS | MEDICATION | CONCERNS |
|---|---|---|
|  |  |  |

My Thoughts and notes

Future Check Up's

_____
_____
_____

IMPORTANT

_____
_____
_____

Date:_____ Patient Name:_____

APPOINTMENT: _____

## Patient Details:
_____
_____
_____
_____

## Patient Histry:
_____
_____
_____
_____

| SYMPTOMS | MEDICATION | CONCERNS |
|---|---|---|
|  |  |  |

### My Thoughts and notes
_____
_____
_____
_____

### Future Check Up's
_____
_____

IMPORTANT
_____
_____

Date:_____ Patient Name:_____

APPOINTMENT: _____

## Patient Details:
_____
_____
_____

## Patient Histry:
_____
_____
_____
_____

| SYMPTOMS | MEDICATION | CONCERNS |
|----------|-----------|----------|
|          |           |          |

### My Thoughts and notes

Future Check Up's
_____
_____

IMPORTANT
_____

Date:_____ Patient Name: _____

APPOINTMENT: _____

## Patient Details:
_____
_____
_____
_____

## Patient Histry:
_____
_____
_____
_____

| SYMPTOMS | MEDICATION | CONCERNS |
|----------|------------|----------|
|          |            |          |

### My Thoughts and notes
_____
_____
_____

### IMPORTANT
_____
_____
_____

### Future Check Up's
_____
_____
_____

Date: _____ Patient Name: _____

APPOINTMENT: _____

## Patient Details:

_____
_____
_____
_____

## Patient Histry:

_____
_____
_____
_____
_____

| SYMPTOMS | MEDICATION | CONCERNS |
|---|---|---|
| | | |

### My Thoughts and notes

Future Check Up's

_____ _____

_____ _____

_____

### IMPORTANT

_____

_____

_____

Date:_____ Patient Name:_____

APPOINTMENT: _____

## Patient Details:
_____
_____
_____
_____

## Patient Histry:
_____
_____
_____
_____

| SYMPTOMS | MEDICATION | CONCERNS |
|---|---|---|
| | | |

### My Thoughts and notes

### Future Check Up's

_____
_____
_____
_____

### IMPORTANT

_____
_____
_____

Date:_____ Patient Name:_____

APPOINTMENT: _____

## Patient Details:

_____
_____
_____
_____

## Patient Histry:

_____
_____
_____
_____
_____

| SYMPTOMS | MEDICATION | CONCERNS |
|---|---|---|
|  |  |  |

### My Thoughts and notes

Future Check Up's

_____
_____
. _____

### IMPORTANT

_____
_____

# Date: _____ Patient Name: _____

APPOINTMENT: _____

## Patient Details:

_____
_____
_____
_____

## Patient Histry:

_____
_____
_____
_____

| SYMPTOMS | MEDICATION | CONCERNS |
|---|---|---|
| | | |

## My Thoughts and notes

Future Check Up's

_____    _____
_____    _____
_____    _____

### IMPORTANT

_____
_____
_____

Date: _____ Patient Name: _____

APPOINTMENT: _____

Patient Details:
_____
_____
_____

Patient Histry:
_____
_____
_____
_____
_____

| SYMPTOMS | MEDICATION | CONCERNS |
|---|---|---|
|  |  |  |

My Thoughts and notes

Future Check Up's

_____
_____
_____
_____

IMPORTANT

_____
_____

# Date:_____ Patient Name: _____

APPOINTMENT: _____

# Patient Details:
_____
_____
_____

# Patient Histry:
_____
_____
_____
_____

| SYMPTOMS | MEDICATION | CONCERNS |
|---|---|---|
| | | |

## My Thoughts and notes

Future Check Up's

_____
_____
_____

### IMPORTANT
_____
_____

Date:_____ Patient Name:_____

APPOINTMENT: _____

## Patient Details:

_____
_____
_____

## Patient Histry:

_____
_____
_____
_____

| SYMPTOMS | MEDICATION | CONCERNS |
|----------|------------|----------|
|          |            |          |

My Thoughts and notes

Future Check Up's

_____
_____
_____

IMPORTANT

_____
_____
_____

Date:_____ Patient Name:_____

APPOINTMENT: _____

## Patient Details:

_____
_____
_____
_____

## Patient Histry:

_____
_____
_____
_____
_____

| SYMPTOMS | MEDICATION | CONCERNS |
|----------|------------|----------|
|          |            |          |

## My Thoughts and notes

_____

### Future Check Up's

_____

**IMPORTANT**

_____

Date:_____ Patient Name:_____

APPOINTMENT: _____

## Patient Details:

_____
_____
_____
_____

## Patient Histry:

_____
_____
_____
_____
_____

| SYMPTOMS | MEDICATION | CONCERNS |
|---|---|---|
|  |  |  |

### My Thoughts and notes

Future Check Up's

_____
_____
_____

### IMPORTANT

_____
_____
_____

Date:_____ Patient Name: _____

APPOINTMENT: _____

## Patient Details:
_____
_____
_____
_____

## Patient Histry:
_____
_____
_____
_____

| SYMPTOMS | MEDICATION | CONCERNS |
|---|---|---|
|  |  |  |

### My Thoughts and notes          Future Check Up's
_____          _____
_____          _____
_____          _____
_____

IMPORTANT
_____
_____
_____

Date:_____ Patient Name:_____

APPOINTMENT: _____

## Patient Details:
_____
_____
_____
_____

## Patient Histry:
_____
_____
_____
_____
_____

| SYMPTOMS | MEDICATION | CONCERNS |
|----------|------------|----------|
|          |            |          |

My Thoughts and notes

Future Check Up's

IMPORTANT

Date: _____ Patient Name: _____

APPOINTMENT: _____

## Patient Details:

_____
_____
_____
_____

## Patient Histry:

_____
_____
_____
_____

| SYMPTOMS | MEDICATION | CONCERNS |
|---|---|---|
|  |  |  |

### My Thoughts and notes

_____
_____
_____

Future Check Up's

_____
_____

### IMPORTANT

_____
_____
_____

Date:_____ Patient Name:_____

APPOINTMENT: _____

## Patient Details:

_____
_____
_____
_____

## Patient Histry:

_____
_____
_____
_____

| SYMPTOMS | MEDICATION | CONCERNS |
|---|---|---|
|  |  |  |

### My Thoughts and notes

_____

### Future Check Up's

_____
_____
_____

### IMPORTANT

_____
_____
_____

# Date: _____ Patient Name: _____

APPOINTMENT: _____

# Patient Details:
_____
_____
_____
_____

# Patient Histry:
_____
_____
_____
_____

| SYMPTOMS | MEDICATION | CONCERNS |
|---|---|---|
|  |  |  |

## My Thoughts and notes
_____
_____
_____
_____

### Future Check Up's
_____
_____

### IMPORTANT
_____
_____
_____

Date:_____ Patient Name:_____

APPOINTMENT: _____

# Patient Details:
_____
_____
_____
_____

# Patient Histry:
_____
_____
_____
_____
_____

| SYMPTOMS | MEDICATION | CONCERNS |
|---|---|---|
|  |  |  |

## My Thoughts and notes
_____

Future Check Up's
_ _ _ _ _ _ _ _ _

_____
_____

## IMPORTANT
_____
_____
_____

Date:_____ Patient Name:_____

APPOINTMENT: _____

Patient Details:
_____
_____
_____
_____

Patient Histry:
_____
_____
_____
_____

| SYMPTOMS | MEDICATION | CONCERNS |
|---|---|---|
| | | |

My Thoughts and notes          Future Check Up's
_____        ........................
_____        ........................
_____        ........................
_____

IMPORTANT
_____
_____
_____
_____

Date:_____ Patient Name:_____

APPOINTMENT: _____

## Patient Details:

_____
_____
_____

## Patient Histry:

_____
_____
_____

| SYMPTOMS | MEDICATION | CONCERNS |
|----------|------------|----------|
|          |            |          |

### My Thoughts and notes

_____
_____
_____

### Future Check Up's

_____

### IMPORTANT

_____
_____
_____

Date: _____ Patient Name: _____

APPOINTMENT: _____

# Patient Details:

_____
_____
_____
_____

# Patient Histry:

_____
_____
_____
_____

| SYMPTOMS | MEDICATION | CONCERNS |
|----------|------------|----------|
|          |            |          |

## My Thoughts and notes

Future Check Up's

_____
_____
_____
_____

IMPORTANT

_____
_____
_____

Date: _____ Patient Name: _____

APPOINTMENT: _____

## Patient Details:
_____
_____
_____

## Patient Histry:
_____
_____
_____
_____

| SYMPTOMS | MEDICATION | CONCERNS |
|---|---|---|
| | | |

### My Thoughts and notes
_____
_____
_____

### Future Check Up's
_____

**IMPORTANT**
_____
_____
_____

Date:_____ Patient Name:_____

APPOINTMENT: _____

## Patient Details:
_____
_____
_____
_____

## Patient Histry:
_____
_____
_____
_____

| SYMPTOMS | MEDICATION | CONCERNS |
|---|---|---|
|  |  |  |

My Thoughts and notes

_____
_____
_____
_____

Future Check Up's

_____
_____
_____

IMPORTANT

_____
_____
_____

Date:_____ Patient Name:_____

APPOINTMENT: _____

Patient Details:
_____
_____
_____

Patient Histry:
_____
_____
_____
_____

| SYMPTOMS | MEDICATION | CONCERNS |
|----------|------------|----------|
|          |            |          |

My Thoughts and notes

Future Check Up's

IMPORTANT

Date:_____ Patient Name:_____

APPOINTMENT: _____

Patient Details:
_____
_____
_____
_____

Patient Histry:
_____
_____
_____
_____

| SYMPTOMS | MEDICATION | CONCERNS |
|---|---|---|
| | | |

My Thoughts and notes

Future Check Up's

_____

_____

_____

IMPORTANT

_____
_____
_____

# Date:_____ Patient Name:_____

APPOINTMENT: _____

## Patient Details:

_____
_____
_____
_____

## Patient Histry:

_____
_____
_____
_____
_____

| SYMPTOMS | MEDICATION | CONCERNS |
|----------|------------|----------|
|          |            |          |

### My Thoughts and notes

_____
_____
_____

### Future Check Up's

.............................
.............................
.............................

### IMPORTANT

_____
_____
_____

Date:_____ Patient Name:_____

APPOINTMENT: _____

## Patient Details:

_____
_____
_____
_____

## Patient Histry:

_____
_____
_____
_____

| SYMPTOMS | MEDICATION | CONCERNS |
|---|---|---|
|  |  |  |

### My Thoughts and notes

### Future Check Up's

_____
_____
_____

**IMPORTANT**

_____
_____
_____

Date: _____ Patient Name: _____

APPOINTMENT: _____

## Patient Details:
_____
_____
_____

## Patient Histry:
_____
_____
_____

| SYMPTOMS | MEDICATION | CONCERNS |
|----------|------------|----------|
|          |            |          |

### My Thoughts and notes
_____
_____

### Future Check Up's
_____

**IMPORTANT**
_____
_____

Date:_____ Patient Name:_____

APPOINTMENT: _____

## Patient Details:

_____
_____
_____
_____

## Patient Histry:

_____
_____
_____
_____

| SYMPTOMS | MEDICATION | CONCERNS |
|----------|------------|----------|
|          |            |          |

## My Thoughts and notes

Future Check Up's

_____    _____
_____    _____
_____    _____

### IMPORTANT

_____
_____
_____

Date:_____ Patient Name:_____

APPOINTMENT: _____

## Patient Details:
_____
_____
_____

## Patient Histry:
_____
_____
_____
_____

| SYMPTOMS | MEDICATION | CONCERNS |
|---|---|---|
|  |  |  |

### My Thoughts and notes
_____
_____
_____

**IMPORTANT**
_____
_____

### Future Check Up's
_____
_____
_____

Date:_____ Patient Name:_____

APPOINTMENT: _____

## Patient Details:
_____
_____
_____
_____

## Patient Histry:
_____
_____
_____
_____

| SYMPTOMS | MEDICATION | CONCERNS |
|----------|------------|----------|
|          |            |          |

## My Thoughts and notes

### Future Check Up's

_____
_____
_____

**IMPORTANT**

Date:_____ Patient Name:_____

APPOINTMENT: _____

## Patient Details:
_____
_____
_____

## Patient Histry:
_____
_____
_____
_____

| SYMPTOMS | MEDICATION | CONCERNS |
| --- | --- | --- |
| | | |

### My Thoughts and notes
_____
_____
_____

**Future Check Up's**
_____
_____

### IMPORTANT
_____
_____
_____

Printed in Great Britain
by Amazon

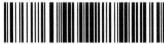
34087162R00070